Intermittent Fasting For Women Over 50

How to Lose Weight and Boost your Energy while Enjoying Amazing and Delicious Recipes

Samantha Thornton

TABLE OF CONTENTS

INTRODUCTION

Obviously, it is necessary to maintain a balanced and healthy diet, rich in vegetables and whole grains and that provides all the macronutrients needed by the body, as well as the right amount of fat (preferably vegetable) and avoid junk food, seasoned and too salty. All in all, however, you can eat anything, even taking a few whims from time to time.

Fasting has positive implications for the health of women over 50. Science has shown that reducing calorie intake prolongs life, because it acts on the metabolic function of longevity genes, reduces senile diseases, cancer, cardiovascular diseases and neurodegenerative ones such as Alzheimer's and Parkinson's disease. In addition, especially for women over 50, it has multiple benefits on mood, fights depression, and contributes to the improvement of energy, libido and concentration. And as if that weren't enough, it gives the skin a better look.

To start this type of "diet" you must first of all be in good health and in any case, before starting, it is always better to consult your doctor. The female body is particularly sensitive to calorie restriction, because the hypothalamus, a gland in the brain responsible for the production of hormones, is stimulated. These hormones risk going haywire with a drastic reduction in calories or too long a fast. The advice is therefore to start gradually, perhaps introducing some vegetable snacks during fasting hours (fennel, lettuce, endive, and radicchio).

As mentioned, in women, intermittent fasting works differently than in men. Sometimes it is more difficult for women to get results. In addition, intermittent fasting on non-consecutive days is better able to keep those annoying hormones under control. Various scientific evidence shows that in order to achieve fat loss, fasting must be tailored to the sex. But there may be variations that allow you to overcome these problems. Fasting can really prove to be a convenient and effective way to optimize your health and make you feel better, but only if it is done in a certain way: the way that is best for each of us.

Fasting, after all, represents the easiest and at the same time powerful detoxification and regeneration therapy that we can offer to cells and the whole organism. Putting certain functions at physiological rest does not, in fact, mean that organs and tissues go into stand-by. On the contrary, thanks to the absence of a continuous metabolic commitment, they can dedicate themselves to something else, activating all those processes of self-repair, catabolism, excretion and cell turnover that only in the absence of nutrients can take place at the highest levels.

At the beginning, and especially the first few times, you don't realize what is happening inside, but it takes very little to feel the effects. Apart from the slight headache that can arise the first time, you usually feel more energetic, concentrated and serene soon. Not only that, the perennial feeling of hunger turns into a pleasant and constant satiety, which is maintained even after returning to normal nutrition.

Another effect of intermittent fasting, especially in overweight women, is to be able - without too much difficulty - to lose weight in the form of adipose tissue. Compared to a chronic low-calorie diet, in fact, an IF protocol can be a much more feasible and effective approach. There are many cases of women who, after trying it, learn to eat well even on feeding days. Obviously, it is not with DIY that lasting results are achieved, and I reiterate that any approach to FH should be planned with the whole dietary context in mind.

In normal weight women, however, the effect on body composition is more unpredictable and controversial. There are those who expect to lose weight but are disappointed because the weight does not vary, and those who notice a better definition, especially in some body areas.

In the first case, it is necessary to understand whether or not the desired weight loss was necessary at the outset, and especially if there are changes in body composition, which is much more important than weight itself. Weight loss, after all, should not be the first or only purpose of intermittent fasting. Some women may also experience morphological changes in their body, such as a thinning waist or a reduction in hip circumference, and this is certainly related to hormonal factors as well as changes in glucidic and insulin metabolism (better insulin sensitivity, less tendency to accumulate visceral fat). These different reactions allow us to make a very important reflection, which concerns the differences between one woman and another in terms of body composition and location of accumulations. For this reason, we must first of all make it clear which objectives we want to achieve and understand that every woman is different from the other.

Each woman is characterized by her own constitutional type and endocrine profile, which determines a wide variability in terms of body composition, glucidic and lipid metabolism, and tendency to accumulate fat in localized areas. Some women with android conformation, for example, localize the largest reserves of adipose tissue at abdominal level, while in gynoid women they more easily concentrate on thighs and buttocks.

It is clear, therefore, that it is useful to assess the suitability of each woman for intermittent fasting according to her body type.

HEALTH AND ESTHETIC BENEFITS OF INTERMITTENT FASTING

Lifestyle Benefits

When compared to other diets, the simplicity of intermittent fasting makes it perhaps the easiest eating protocol through which to experience significant health benefits. Often, the complexity of some eating plans causes people to fail at the first hurdle because as much as they think they understand what they should be doing, they really don't. This results in people going to punishing extremes in order to fulfill what they think they are supposed to be doing and ending up with very disappointing results. Intermittent fasting couldn't be simpler—now you eat and now you don't. Often, special diets can be extremely expensive to follow. You have to purchase special ingredients and eat food that you ordinarily wouldn't. Intermittent fasting is different in that regard too. It costs you absolutely nothing to practice intermittent fasting, and other than a caloric reduction in the case of weight loss and eating as healthy as possible, there is no dictation as to what to eat.

Intermittent fasting is flexible, so it allows you gaps in between to eat the things you enjoy. What is life without an occasional dessert, some chocolate, or pizza? With intermittent fasting, you can have those treats and not feel guilty because when you fast, your body will be burning that treat off. Of course, that is not to say that in every eating window you can binge on every fast food known to mankind. You will still need to eat a healthy diet; you just won't be weighing food and calculating its calorie content all the time.

If you have found an eating plan that you enjoy such as Keto, Paleo, or the like, you can incorporate that with intermittent fasting. There are no other plans available where you can combine two and get even better results. Intermittent fasting is a fantastic addition to other eating plans and does not detract from any other diets (Fung, 2020).

For women over 50, the adjustment to menopause can mean a temporary change in lifestyle. In severe situations, menopause can result in difficulties in relationships with partners and loved ones. Intermittent fasting can help make a big difference in these challenges, and this can be life-changing.

Health Benefits

Cardiovascular health should be a strong focus for people of all ages but even more so for women over 50. The most significant cause of death for women over 50 today is cardiovascular disease. This umbrella term describes all diseases of the heart or the arteries leading to and from the heart. This could include blockages, damage, and deformities in structure. There are several risk factors that contribute to the occurrence of cardiovascular disease including smoking, physical inactivity, genetics, and diet. The latter, however, has been found to be the largest controllable contributor to heart disease.

The most impactful factor where diet is concerned is the types of protein sources that are eaten as well as the types of fats that are consumed. Plant proteins such as beans and legumes have been proven to be a healthier source of protein than animal proteins in general.

Where animal protein is concerned, the leaner the source, the better, and poultry and fish are always healthier options than red meat. The fat component of red meat is another problem where heart disease is concerned, as are other sources of fat such as cooking oils and spreads used for bread. Saturated fats are the types of fats we want to avoid in our diet, and these include animal fat, lard, and tropical oils such as palm oil. Unsaturated fats in small quantities are healthier. Examples of unsaturated fats include avocados, nuts, olive oil, and vegetable oils. When we eat foods in excess of what our body is able to burn, the leftover food forms triglycerides that, at high levels, contribute to the occurrence of cardiovascular disease. When we fast, our body burns triglycerides for energy thereby reducing the levels in our blood and, in turn, reducing our risk of cardiovascular disease.

This decrease in insulin results in less food being stored as fat. In animal trials, intermittent fasting has been shown to prevent and reverse Type 2 Diabetes. Another thing that happens when insulin levels decrease is that the FOXO transcription factors, which are known to positively impact metabolism, become more active in the body. This process is also linked to improved longevity and healthy aging.

Another no communicable disease that seems to be impacted by intermittent fasting is cancer. Growth Factor 1 (GF1) is a hormone very similar in nature to insulin, and the presence of this hormone is known to be a marker for cancer development. Levels of GF1 are reduced during intermittent fasting. Women over 50 are twice as likely to develop breast cancer, for instance, and risk factors for other common cancers are also thought to increase when women start to experience the hormonal changes of menopause. Intermittent fasting is, therefore, an excellent preventative measure for the occurrence of cancer in women over 50.

The increased cell resilience seen in people who regularly fast has been linked to a stronger immune system as well as general faster recovery from illness. The process of building cell resilience through fasting is similar to exercising muscles. The more you undertake regular exercise with periods of rest in between, the stronger your muscles become.

The autophagy process that is triggered by intermittent fasting has been shown to help reduce inflammation in the body as well as oxidative stress, which is primarily responsible for cell damage in the body. Inflammation in various parts of the body has been shown to be present as a precursor to the diagnosis of many different no communicable diseases. The diagnosis of no communicable diseases is far more common in women over 50 than any other age group. It is, therefore, vital for women in this age group to make use of intermittent fasting and autophagy as an additional preventative measure against the development of no communicable diseases.

The Circadian Cycle is the name given to the rhythm created in our body by light and dark (day and night). This natural rhythm controls our need to sleep and eat and has a major impact on our metabolism, cognitive function, and emotional health. It is our internal clock, and when disrupted, it can have devastating effects on our bodies. Intermittent fasting has been shown to help regulate the Circadian Cycle and, if it is out of loop, reset it back to its natural function.

From an evolutionary perspective, our bodies are designed to eat during the day and not to eat at night. This, of course, is the reverse in certain nocturnal mammals who have evolved to reverse that Circadian Cycle due to the availability of prey at night. As modern humans, we have disrupted our Circadian Cycle by not going to sleep when the sun goes down and also continuing to eat well into the night. This impacts our metabolism and our sleeping patterns, resulting in weight gain and sleep disorders such as insomnia. By using intermittent fasting to reset our internal clock to its evolutionary default, we can encourage weight loss by optimizing our metabolism and have a more restful sleep.

In women over 50, this is particularly beneficial. As we age, sleep disorders become more common. We feel tired earlier, experience disturbed sleep, and generally find that we are unable to sleep for as many hours as we once could. This disruption in sleep, of course, has a major impact on our health both physically and mentally. The reason for this change in sleep is due to the reduced levels of Human Growth Hormone (HGH) in our bodies as we age. As we now know, intermittent fasting helps to increase the levels of HGH in our body, thus allowing us to regain a more regular sleeping pattern.

If you eat too long before you go to bed, you may experience hunger pangs while you sleep that disrupt your sleep. If you eat too large a meal before going to sleep, your body will still be diverting additional blood flow to your stomach to digest its contents, and that will also disrupt your sleep. The importance of a good sleeping pattern cannot be understated as poor sleeping patterns have even been shown to increase the likelihood of the occurrence of certain cancers.

Intermittent fasting has also been shown to improve the regulation of genes that promote liver health and also in the balance of gut bacteria. Gut bacteria play a role in our immune system, and it is vital to keep these gut guests in good shape to optimize your body's defense systems (Kresser, 2019).

<u>Cognitive Functioning Benefits</u>

As you move into your 50s, there are several different effects on your brain health and, as a result, your cognitive functioning. Brain shrinkage automatically occurs as we age, and although it is not something we can avoid, it is certainly something that we can delay and slow down. From a fasting perspective, the process of autophagy, which speeds up during fasting, can help to consume damaged brain cells and use that cellular material to produce new brain cells. This process can help to alleviate the natural brain shrinkage process.

The release of ketones during the burning of fat which occurs during fasting is also highly beneficial to brain health. The enhanced level of ketones helps to protect the brain from the development of epileptic seizures, Alzheimer's disease, and other neurodegenerative diseases. Of course, as we age, we are also more likely to develop neurodegenerative diseases. Diseases like Alzheimer's and other forms of dementia do have a wide range of risk factors including genetics and smoking. Fasting to enhance autophagy and ketone production is one way that we put up a line of defense against these diseases.

Intermittent fasting can also help to improve neuroplasticity, which is the brain's natural capability to build new neural pathways. This is imperative in learning as well as in the breaking of habits. When we break bad habits, we actually work to remove the brain's reliance on a commonly used neural pathway and promote the use of a new pathway. Studies in people with brain injuries have shown that intermittent fasting speeds up healing.

GUIDELINES TO START YOUR INTERMITTENT FASTING

How to fast safely
Since there are so many risks involving intermittent fasting, it is important to take precautionary measures and opt for a safe road to achieving all its benefits. The following measures can help women of all ages, especially those over 50, to fast without causing any damage to their physical and mental health.

Choose the Right Method
Intermittent fasting works differently for everyone, as the metabolic rates differ from one person to another. Just jumping into a routine, knowing only the benefits, can be dangerous. Women in this age group are advised to have a checkup first, calculate their body mass index and weight, look for any other health problems, and then choose a particular fasting method. Fasting every day might not help women who are diabetic. In this case they must fast only for a short duration and with wider gaps to maintain their health. Start slow, then gradually increase the duration of the fast as the body adapts to the new regime.

Nutritional Needs
Most women opt for intermittent fasting only to lose weight. In the weight loss struggle, they may turn a blind eye on their nutritional needs. Fasting does not mean depriving the body of what it needs to function properly. Therefore, meeting nutritional needs is imperative in this regard. Consume all the macro and micronutrients in your diet. Fibers, vitamins, minerals, phytonutrients are as important as proteins, carbohydrates, and fats for optimal brain and body function. The meal before and after the fast should be rich in quality, containing a wide range of nutrients.

Eating is Essential
Do not go for a fasting method that would cause intense hunger pangs. Start off with a short duration fast by adding a few hours to your normal gaps between the two meals. Eating is as essential as the fast itself. A complete abstention from food can result in malnutrition, so eat good and healthy food.

Hydrate

When the body is in the fasting state, it goes in ketosis. Loss of water through increased urination is the direct outcome of ketosis. Dehydration can lead to electrolyte imbalance in the body. Therefore, it is very important to constantly hydrate yourself. During the fast, women can drink water, zero-calorie juices and drinks to maintain the natural water levels of the body. Two to three liters of water consumption in a day are necessary when you are on intermittent fasting.

Steadily Break the Fast

You may feel a predilection to eat everything at once when you break the fast. But this is an unhealthy act. Providing excessive nutrients to a fasted body at a time may lead to obesity and lethargy. It will reverse all the good effects of the fast. So, break your fast slowly by consuming small meals after every half an hour during the FED state. Do not rely on a single meal; break it into several meals, ranging in flavors and ingredients to meet your nutritional needs. For instance, break your fast with a glass of smoothie, then leave a gap and follow with a protein-rich meal full of grains, fruits, and vegetables.

No Overeating

Breaking the fast does not mean you can start stuffing your body with every edible item. Overeating is still harmful to a fasting regime. Remember, the goal of fasting is to restrict caloric consumption, and overeating does not help to achieve it. Therefore, avoid binge eating after the fast and eat just enough to meet the body's basic needs of energy, vitamins, mineral, and fibers.

Balanced Meals

A balanced meal contains high doses of protein and controlled amounts of fats along with smaller amounts of carbs, paired with traces of minerals, vitamins, and fibers. Whatever you eat before or after the fast, make sure to maintain this balance. For example, if you are cooking a delicious steak for your meal, then add some sautéed vegetables or whole grains, a drizzle of olive oil, some grated cheese, nuts, and seeds.

Switch between Time Periods

There is no fixed formula to fast! There are several methods to choose from, and a person can switch from one method to another, depending on the changes they are experiencing. As women over 50 are constantly going into hormonal and physical changes, they can turn to other methods of fasting if the method they are following isn't working for their health. Your fasting regime should only be health-centric; it doesn't have to be tied to a specific number of hours or days.

Work Out

Most women over the age of 50 start considering themselves too old to exercise as they experience weakening of bones and lowering of the metabolism. But exercise is proved to be crucial in harnessing the benefits of a fast and a healthy diet. But it is recommended for women in their 50s not to over exhaust themselves during the fasting state. Only 10 to 15 minutes of light exercises are enough to keep you fit and active.

Monitor the Changes

Without keeping track of the changes that your body experiences after fasting, you can't really maintain a healthy routine. Women in their 50s should look out for any sign of discomfort or other symptoms during the fast which are considered harmful. Monitor the blood sugar levels, hunger levels, change in body weight and improvement in health conditions to keep track of the progress.

How to break the fast? Tips & tricks to break your fast

The way a person breaks the fast is as important as the fast itself. No matter which of the above-mentioned methods of fasting a person chooses, without consuming a healthy meal with balanced nutrients, the real benefits of a fasting regime cannot be achieved. Remember, the main aim of intermittent fasting is weight loss and boosting the metabolic rate in order to fight against several health problems. If the fast is not paired with a healthy diet, it will not lead to desirable results. It is actually the case with many people who complain about the inefficiency of intermittent fasting. When people opt for the fasting regime, they focus solely on the fasting state, and once that stage is over, they believe all the work is done; however, that is far from reality. The FED state of the fasting regime is much more important and should be controlled with much care and proper planning.

When the body goes into fasting state, it experiences several gradual changes. The glucose levels reduce gradually as the fast goes on. Initially, when we break the fast, the body reacts by storing energy in the form of fats more than usual to prevent any future deprivation. And when the body receives more calories than its immediate energy needs it will store the excess, thus leading to obesity. Therefore, it is imperative to consume a healthy and proportionate meal to avoid calorie excess accumulation.

Have you ever felt dull and lethargic right after breaking the fast? That is commonly observed by people who usually fast. It is not the fast that actually makes a person feel low; rather, it is the meal after the fast which causes it. That is why intermittent fasting requires a healthy diet. The following considerations must be kept in mind before breaking the fast.

Go Slow

It is true that the meal consumed between the two consecutive fasting periods should be rich enough to meet the body's nutritional needs, but overconsumption should be avoided at a time. Every person has his own metabolic pace, and the body only utilizes a portion of the meal depending on the needs. As the excess is stored as fats, no one should consume more than the body can use. When you break the fast, go slow on the meal and gradually add meals to the FED state. After a long duration fast, there is not much time left to have multiple meals, so people try to have everything at once. There is no harm in eating one big meal, but the FED state should not start with this heavy meal.

Think of the FED state as a multi-course meal; the more the courses, the healthier it will be. Start with an appetizer to break the fast. Give your body some time to process those calories and gain the minimum required energy. Such appetizers do not have to be high carb meals, but fresh and organic food should be consumed as stated above.

About 1 or 2 hours after the first appetizer, go for a more proper meal, which can be anything ranging from soups, stews, grilled steaks, seafood, satays, etc. This meal should be filled with a wide range of nutrients; you can always add a side dish like salads or dips, etc. When you are done with this meal, give your body a break for 4-5 hours until you will have the next meal, right before the fast. There can be two or three meals between the two consecutive fasting periods, depending on how long the fast lasts. Intake of juices and water must remain constant during this time.

Avoid Binge Eating

Binge eating is defined as uncontrolled consumption of food, and when a person breaks a fast, it may push him to binge eat all types of food just to satisfy the cravings. When you have low blood glucose levels, it leads to more cravings and vigorous eating. It is hard to resist for those who are already suffering from binge eating disorders.

Eric Stice, Kendra Davis, Nicole P. Miller, and C. Nathan Marti studied the relation between binge eating and fasting. The study was conducted on 496 participants who were put on the fasting regime. About 23 percent of the participants showed a prominent sign of binge eating tendency and bulimia nervosa. The study concluded that people who fast can develop the tendency of binge eating more than people who are on other calorie restriction diet plans. Thus, people who fast need to fight against tendencies to binge eating. Breaking one single meal into multiple meals or adding more side dishes and snacks to the FED state of the fasting regime can help you resist the craving for excessive food consumption. Keep a constant intake of low or zero-calorie beverages all the time; this will prevent the urge to eat. Use fillers like leafy green vegetables and low carb fruits to cope with food cravings. Remember, the whole fasting program is designed to restrict the daily or weekly caloric intake, and binge eating during the FED state can make this goal unachievable. So, while you restrict food during the fasting period, you must also avoid over consumption when breaking the fast.

HOW INTERMITTENT FASTING WORK

Intermittent fasting is the technique of scheduling your dishes for your body to obtain the most out of them. Rather than minimizing your calorie use in fifty percent, refuting yourself of all the foods you value, or diving right into a classy diet plan pattern, Intermittent fasting is an all-natural, logical, as well as healthy and balanced and also balanced method of eating that advertises fat burning. There are tons of ways to approach Intermittent Fasting.

It's defined as an eating pattern. This technique focuses on altering when you take in, instead of what you consume.

When you begin Intermittent fasting, you will be more than likely to maintain your calorie intake the same; nonetheless, in contrast to spreading your dishes throughout the day, you will undoubtedly eat more significant recipes throughout a much shorter amount of time. As opposed to consuming 3 to 4 meals a day, you might eat one big meal at 11 am, afterward an added large dish at 6 pm, without any dine-in between 11 am as well as 6 pm, as well as also after 6 pm, no meal up until 11 am the adhering to day. This is simply one strategy of recurring fasting, and likewise, others will be examined in this book in later stages.

Intermittent Fasting is a technique used by whole lots of bodybuilders, specialist athletes, and also physical health and fitness masters to maintain their muscular tissue mass high and their body fat percent reduced. Recurring fasting can be done short term or long term, but the very best results originate from embracing this technique right into your everyday lifestyle.

The word "fasting" might stress the average person; intermittent fasting does not associate with starving yourself. To comprehend the principals behind effective Intermittent fasting, we'll at first review the body's digestion state: the fed state as well as the fasting state.

For 3 to 5 hours after consuming a meal, your body remains in what is described as the "fed state." Throughout the fed state, your insulin levels rise to soak up and digest your meal. When your insulin levels get high, it is exceptionally tough for your body to shed fat. Insulin is a hormone produced by the pancreatic to handle sugar degrees in the bloodstream. Its purpose is to manage insulin is technically a hormonal storage agent. When insulin degrees come to be so high, your body starts shedding your food for energy instead of your conserved fat. Which is why boosted degrees of it protect against weight reduction.

After the 3 to 5 hrs. are up, your body has, in fact, finished refining the dish, and also you enter the post-absorptive state. The post-absorptive state lasts anywhere from 8 to 12 hours. When your body comes, hereafter the time room is the fasted state. As a result of the reality that your body has refined your food by this.

Factor, your insulin levels are reduced, making you kept fat extremely available for losing.

Persisting fasting allows your body to get to an innovative weight loss state that you would usually obtain to with the average' 3 meals daily' eating pattern. They are just altering the timing as well as the pattern of their food intake. It may take some time to get when you start an Intermittent Fasting program right into the swing of points. Merely obtain back if you slip up right into your Intermittent fasting pattern when you can.

Making a way of living adjustment entails a purposeful initiative, and also no one expects you to do it completely today. Intermittent fasting will definitely take some getting used to if you are not in the practice of going long periods without eating. As long as you pick the right technique for you, continue to be focused, and also remain concentrated, you will unanimously grasp it quickly.

Unlike some of the other diet regimen strategy that you may embark on, the Intermittent fast is one that will certainly work. When you listen to, it is simple to obtain a bit terrified regarding fasting.

Recurring fasting is a little bit various than you might assume. If you finish up being on, your body will often go right into hunger mode, the rapid for as well lengthy.

You do not need to get as well concerned about exactly how this Intermittent quickly will work in the cravings mode. The Intermittent fast is efficient because you are not going too quickly for as long that the body gets in right into this malnourishment setting as well as stops minimizing weight. Instead, it will make the rapid continue long enough that you will have the ability to accelerate the metabolic process.

With the Intermittent quick, you will discover that when you opt for a couple of hrs. Without eating (usually no more than 2 - 4 hrs.), the body is not going to go right into malnourishment setting. When complying with a recurring fasting plan, you require your body to melt more fat without placing in any sort-of extra job.

Here are a couple of fast pointers for success:

Mostly, it is essential not to expect to see outcomes from your new lifestyle promptly. Perhaps, you need to focus on devoting to the process for a minimum of 30 days before you can start to evaluate the results correctly.

Second, it is imperative to remember that the excellent quality of the food you place into your body still matters as it will certainly merely take a few convenience food meals to reverse all of your tough work.

For the excellent results, you will plan to consist of an in-light exercise routine during quick days along with a far more fundamental regimen for full-calorie days.

Recurring Fasting describes nutritional consuming patterns that include not consuming or continues limiting calories for a long-term period, Intermittent Fasting (. There are various subgroups of regular fasting each with variance in the duration of the fast of individuals, some for hrs. others for day(s). This has finished up being an extremely liked subject in the clinical research area as a result of every one of the prospective advantages of fitness in addition to health that is being found.

The diet regimen you adhere to whilst Recurring Fasting will be figured out by the results that you are looking for as well as where you are beginning with additionally, so take a look at on your own and ask the question what do I want from this?

If you are looking for to lose a significant quantity of weight, then you are misting likely to have to take a look at your diet regimen plan extra closely, yet if you wish to shed a couple of pounds for the beach, then you could discover that a pair of weeks of Recurring fasting can do that for you.

There are many various ways you can do recurring fasting. We just are most likely to consider the 24-hour fasting system in which is what I used to shed 27 pounds over a 2-month duration. You could really feel some cravings pains, but these will pass also, as you end up being even more familiar with Intermittent fasting you might find as I have that feeling of need no more existing you with a concern.

If you are fretted that you are not getting adequate nutrients into your body, then you might consider a juice made from celery, lime, broccoli, and also ginger, which will taste fantastic and also get some sufficient nutrient fluid into your body. It would be best to stick to the coffee, water, and tea if you can handle it.

Whatever your diet strategy is whether it's healthy or not you should see weight reduction after regarding three weeks of Intermittent Fasting as well as do not be put off if you do not find much advancement at first, it's not a race, and also it is much far better to drop weight in a straight style over time as opposed to collision losing a couple of extra pounds which you will put right back on. After the initial month, you might want to have an appearance at your diet plan on non-fasting days and also remove high sugar foods and even any scrap that you might generally take in. I have discovered that intermittent fasting over the long-term tends to make me wish to consume healthier foods as an all-natural routine.

If you are practicing intermittent fasting for bodybuilding, then you may wish to consider having a look at your macro-nutrients and also working out just how much healthy protein as well as carbohydrate you call for to eat, this is a lot more complex, as well as you can uncover info about this on several websites which you will need to spend time examining for the very best end results.

There are great deals of advantages to recurring fasting, which you will view as you proceed, a few of these advantages include even more energy, much less bloating, a clearer mind, and a basic feeling of wellness. It's important not to succumb to any type of lure to binge eat after a fasting duration, as this will negate the influence obtained from the recurring fasting period.

In verdict simply by adhering to a two times a week 24-hour Intermittent Fasting approach for a couple of weeks you will slim down however if you can boost your diet plan on the days that you do not rapid then you will lose more weight and if you can remain with this system, then you will certainly keep the weight off without turning to any kind of fad diet regimen or diet plans that are difficult to stick to.

INTERMITTENT FASTING TYPES

There are countless types of intermittent fasting. There are so many reasons why decide to follow an intermittent fasting lifestyle, and at least as many methods for doing it. Therefore, it is fundamental to set some basic definitions before we go deep in detail.

Fasting – Giving up the intake of food or anything that has calories for a particular time frame. Normally, some non-caloric beverages and water are allowed.

Intermittent Fasting – To fast intermittently by adding fasts into your regular meal plan.

Extended Fasting – Fasting for a drawn-out time. It will, in general, be cultivated for a significant long time.

Time-Restricted Feeding – Restricting your regular food usage inside a particular time window. This is meant to improve circadian rhythm and general wellness.

Generally, people who do intermittent fasting restrict their eating time and increase their fasting time. To have something like an actual fast, it would need to prop up for over 24 hours since that is the spot most of the benefits start to kick in.

First, let's have an overview of 10 of the main types of intermittent fasting, then we'll go deep into the 6 that better suit women after 50.

24-Hour Fasting

It is the fundamental technique of intermittent fasting—you fast for around 24 hours, and a short time later has a meal. Despite what the name may suggest, you won't actually go through an entire day without eating. Simply eat around the evening, fast all through the next day, and then eat again in the evening.

You can even have your food at the 23-hour check and eat it inside an hour. The idea is to make a very prominent caloric shortage for the day. Most of the benefits will be vain if you, regardless of fasting, binge and put on weight during the eating time frame.

Gradually and occasionally, you can decide to fast according to your physical condition and needs of the moment.

A fit person who works out constantly would require more eating time frames and a few fasting periods.

An overweight person who is sedentary and needs to lose some more weight could follow an intermittent fasting plan as long as they can until they lose the overabundance weight.

16/8 Intermittent Fasting

Martin Berkhan of Lean gains defined 16:8 intermittent fasting. It is used for improving fat loss while not having to go through an extremely demanding process.

You fast for 16 hours and eat your food inside 8. What number of meals you have inside that time length is irrelevant, yet whatever it is recommended to keep them around 2-3.

In my opinion, this should be the base fasting length to concentrate on reliably by everybody. There is no physical need to eat any sooner than that, and the restriction has many benefits.

Many people think it is more straightforward to postpone breakfast by two or three hours and then eat the last meal around early evening. You should not get insane, and it is demanding to observe the fast. The idea is simply to reduce the proportion of time we spend in an eating state and fast for a large portion of the day.

The Warrior Diet

Ori Hofmekler proposes the Warrior Diet. He talks about the benefits of fasting on blood pressure through hormesis.

During daylight, they used to stroll around with 40 pounds of armor, build fortresses, and bear the hot sun of the Mediterranean, while having just a quick bite. They would have a huge supper around evening time consisting of stews, meat, bread, and many other things.

In the Warrior Diet, you fast for around 20 hours, have a short high power workout, and eat your food during a 4 hours window. Overall, it would merge either two minor meals with a break or one single huge supper.

One Meal a Day OMAD

One Meal a Day Diet, also called OMAD, simply consists of eating just one big meal every day
With OMAD, you regularly fast around 21-23 hours and eat your food inside a 1-2 hour time slot. This is remarkable for dieting since you can feel full and satisfied once the eating time comes.
It is unmatched for losing fat; be that as it may, not ideal for muscle improvement because of time for protein production and anabolism.

36-Hour Fasting

In the past, people would quite commonly go a couple of days without eating; they probably suffered and yet even thrived. Today, the average person can't bear to skip breakfast or go to bed hungry.
For over 24 hours is the spot where all the magic begins; the more you stay in a fasted state and experience hardship, the more your body is forced to trigger its supply systems that start to draw on fat stores, bolster rejuvenating microorganisms, and reuse old wrecked cell material through the system of autophagy.
It takes, at any rate, an entire day to see significant signs of autophagy. Yet, you can speed it up by eating low carb before starting the fast, rehearsing on an unfilled stomach, and drinking some homemade teas that facilitate the challenge.
For 36 hours, it's not really that annoying. You fundamentally eat the night before, don't eat anything during the day, go to sleep on an empty stomach, then wake up the next day, fast a few more hours, and begin eating again.
To make the fasting more straightforward, there are mineral water, plain coffee, green tea, and some homemade teas.

48-Hour Fasting

In case you made it to the 36-hour mark, why not give it a try to fast for a straight 48 hours.
It is only annoying getting through the change of habits. Once you overcome this obstacle, which generally occurs around your usual dinnertime, it gets a lot more straightforward.

The moment your body goes into an increasingly significant ketosis phase and autophagy starts, you will overcome hunger, feel very mentally clear, and have greater mindfulness and focus.

The most problematic bit of any complete fast is around the 24-hour mark. If you can make it to fall asleep and wake up the next day, you have set yourself prepared for fasting for a significant time with no issues from that moment onward. You essentially need to get over this hidden obstacle.

Going to bed hungry sounds disturbing; in any case, this is what a huge part of the world's population does daily. This could make you think about your own luck and feel thankful for having food anytime you want.

Expanded Fasting (3-7 Days)

48-hours fasting would give you a short ride in autophagy and some fat consumption. To genuinely get the deep health benefits of fasting, you would have to fast for three or more days.

It has been shown that 72-hours of fasting can reset the immune system in mice. However, studies on humans have not confirmed that conclusion; also, there may be some issues in prolonged fasting that are not under severe medical control.

Three to five days is the perfect time frame for autophagy, after which you may begin to see unwanted losses in bulk and muscle. Fasting for seven or more days is not generally suggested. Most people do not need to fast any longer than that since it may make them lose muscle tissue.

Fit people may want to focus on three-four of these expanded fasts every year, to propel cell recovery and clean out the body. Notwithstanding a healthy eating routine without any junk food, I do it anyway four times a year because of their tremendous benefits.

In case you are overweight or experience the negative effects of some illness, then longer fasts can really help you get back in health. Fast for three to five days, have a little refreshment break and repeat the plan until needed. I'll never say that enough; if you decide to go through this kind of longer fasting, be always sure of what you are doing and consult a doctor for any doubt.

Alternate Day Fasting

Alternate Day Fasting, as for the 5:2 Diet, is a very common type of fasting. Are they fully considered fasting, despite allowing the intake of 500/660 calories a day on fasting days? Well, yes, they are, since these limited amounts of calories are only intended to help extend perseverance.

To have a sporadic caloric intake will not enable the whole of the physiological benefits of fasting to fully manifest. It would limit a part of the effect. In any case, a strict limitation is important for both your physiology and mind.

Everybody can fast. It is just that someone cannot psychologically bear the weight of not eating. Fasting mimicking diets and alternate-day fasting in this respect.

Fasting Mimicking Diet (FMD)

The Fasting Mimicking Diet can be used every so often. Commonly, people who cannot actually fast, like old people or some recovering patients follow it.

Fasting mimicking diet has been shown to reduce blood pressure, lower insulin, and cover IGF-1, all of which have positive life length benefits. Regardless, these effects are likely an immediate consequence of the huge caloric restriction.

During the Fasting Mimicking Diet, you would eat low protein, moderate carb, and moderate fat foods like mushroom soup, olives, kale wafers, and some nut bars. The idea is to give you something to eat while keeping the calories as low as reasonable. In most cases, again, this is more about satisfying people's psychological needs of eating than the physical ones.

With zero calories would be just as effective, and it would keep up more muscle tissue by increasingly significant ketosis. To thwart the unwanted loss of lean mass, you can adapt the macronutrient taken in during Fasting Mimicking Diet and make them more ketogenic by cutting down the carbs and increasing the fats.

Protein Sparing Modified Fasting

Protein-Sparing Modified Fast (PSMF) is a low carb, low fat, high protein type of diet that helps to get increasingly fit quite fast while keeping muscle toned.

Lean mass is a significant matter of stress for healthy people, especially in case they are endeavoring to do intermittent fasting.

A catabolic stressor will, over the long term, lead to muscle loss; notwithstanding, the loss rate is a lot lower than people may imagine. To prevent that from happening, you have to stay in ketosis and lower the body's appetite for glucose.

PSMF is absolutely going to keep up more muscle than the fasting-mimicking diet. Yet, there's the danger of staying out of ketosis in case you are already eating many proteins preparing yourself for muscle catabolism.

BREAKFASTS RECIPE

1. <u>Broccoli Rabe with Lemon and Cheese</u>

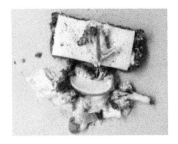

Preparation Time: 5 minutes

Cooking Time: 15 minutes

Servings: 4

Ingredients:

- 1 quart of Water 1 teaspoon of Salt
- ½ cup of Broccoli rabe, trimmed
- 2 tablespoons of Olive oil
- 2 cloves of Garlic, chopped
- 1 tablespoon of Lemon juice
- Salt Pepper
- 2 tablespoons of Parmesan cheese

Directions:

1. Boil water; add salt and broccoli rabe. On low heat, simmer for about 8 minutes. Drain and shock under cold water and dry on paper towels.

2. Heat olive oil over medium-low heat and sauté the garlic for 5 minutes. Cut the broccoli rabe stems into 2 pieces and add to the garlic and olive oil. Sprinkle with lemon juice, salt, and pepper. Serve the Parmesan cheese at the table.

Nutrition: Calories 81 kcal Fat 8 g Protein 2 g Carbs 2 g

2. Cauliflower Fried Rice

Preparation Time: 10 minutes

Cooking Time: 10 minutes

Servings: 5

Ingredients:

- 1 Cauliflower head, halved
- 2 tablespoons of Sesame oil
- 2 Onions, chopped
- 1 Egg, beaten
- 5 tablespoons of coconut aminos

Directions:

1. Place a steam rack in the Instant Pot and add a cup of water.
2. Place the cauliflower florets on the steam rack.
3. Set the lid in place and the vent to point to "Sealing."
4. Press the "Steam" button and adjust the time to 7 minutes.
5. Release the pressure quickly.
6. In a food processor, add in cauliflower florets and pulse until grainy in texture.
7. Sauté the oil.
8. Stir in the onions until fragrant.
9. Stir in the egg and break it up into small pieces.
10. Add the cauliflower rice and season with coconut aminos.
11. Add in more pepper and salt if desired.

Nutrition: Calories 108 kcal Carbs 4.3 g Protein 3.4 g Fat 8.2 g

3. <u>Avocado Deviled Eggs</u>

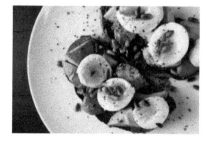

Preparation Time: 10 minutes

Cooking Time: 6 minutes

Servings: 6

Ingredients:

- 6 Eggs

- 1 Avocado, pitted and meat scooped

- ¼ teaspoon of Garlic powder

- ¼ teaspoon of Paprika, smoked

- 3 tablespoons of Cilantro, chopped

Directions:

1. Place the eggs in the Instant Pot and add 1½ cups of water.

2. Close the lid and make sure that the vent points to "Sealing."

3. Select the "Manual" option and cook for 6 minutes.

4. Do quick pressure and release.

5. Allow the eggs to completely cool before cracking and peeling off the shells.

6. Beat the eggs and remove the yolk.

7. In a bowl, mix the yolk, paprika, avocado, and garlic powder. Sprinkle with pepper and salt.

8. Stuff the avocado-yolk mixture into the hollow egg whites.

9. Garnish with cilantro.

Nutrition: Calories 184 kcal Carbs 4.1 g Protein 9.6 g Fat 14.5 g

4. Fresh Fig and Raspberry Compote

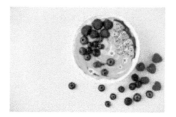

Preparation Time: 3 minutes

Cooking Time: 17 minutes

Servings: 4

Ingredients:

- ½ cup of Honey
- ¼ cup of Water
- 12 Mission figs, ripe
- 1 cup of Red raspberries
- 1 tablespoon of mint leaves, freshly chopped

Directions:

1. Mix honey and water together in a glass bowl and microwave on high for 20 seconds. Remove, stir, and let chill in the refrigerator.
2. Cut the figs into quarters and add them to the chilled honey syrup.
3. Add the raspberries and mint to the chilled syrup and let sit for 15 minutes in the refrigerator.
4. To serve, scoop the figs and raspberries onto four dessert plates.

Nutrition: Calories 242 kcal Fat 1 g Protein 2 g Carbs 62 g

5. Oven-Roasted Pears

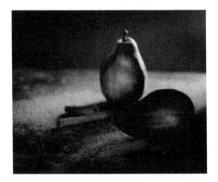

Preparation Time: 6 minutes

Cooking Time: 55 minutes

Servings: 4

Ingredients:

- 4 Bosc pears, ripe
- 1½ cups of Marsala wine

Directions:

1. Preheat oven to 450°F.

2. Place pears upright in a baking dish and pour the Marsala wine over them. Bake the pears for 20 minutes. Add water or more Marsala if the dish starts to get dry.

3. Baste the pears with the liquid in the dish and bake 20 minutes more.

4. Baste the pears again and bake longer until a knife inserted in a pear goes in easily.

5. Take out the pears and baste them several times as they cool. Serve at room temperature with a knife and fork.

Nutrition: Calories 217 kcal Fat 0.5 g Protein 1 g Carbs 31 g

6. Hawaiian-style Snow Cones

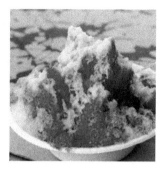

Preparation Time: 5 minutes

Cooking Time: 5 minutes

Servings: 4

Ingredients:

- 4 tablespoons of Red bean paste
- 4 small scoops of Vanilla ice cream
- 4 cups of Shaved ice
- ½ cup of Syrup, flavored for snow cones

Directions:

1. Place a tablespoon of sweet red bean paste in the bottom of four insulated paper cones or cups.
2. Top the sweet red bean paste with a scoop of vanilla ice cream in each cone or cup.
3. Put a cup of shaved ice on top of the vanilla ice cream in each cone or cup.
4. Drizzle 2 tablespoons of flavored syrup over each shaved ice mound. Serve immediately.

Nutrition: Calories 259 kcal Fat 7 g Protein 3 g Carbs 48 g

7. Vanilla Yogurt

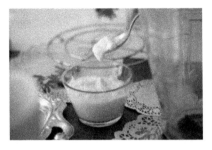

Preparation Time: 10 hours

Cooking Time: 6 hours

Servings: 6

Ingredients:

- ½ gallon of Milk
- ½ cup of Yogurt starter
- ½ cup of Erythritol
- 1 tablespoon of Vanilla extract, pure
- 1 cup of Heavy cream

Directions:

1. Pour the milk into a crockpot and turn it on low for 3 hours.
2. Whisk in vanilla, heavy cream, and Erythritol and let the yogurt set.
3. While on low, cook for about 3 hours.
4. Whisk in your yogurt starter in 1 cup of milk. Add to the crockpot and mix well.
5. Set the lid in place and wrap the crockpot using two beach towels.

6. Let your wrapped crockpot sit for 10 hours while the yogurt cultures.

Nutrition: Calories 256 kcal Fat 21 g Carbs 6 g Protein 4 g

8. Banana Fritters

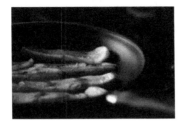

Preparation Time: 10 minutes

Cooking Time: 8 minutes

Servings: 2

Ingredients:

- ¼ cup of Almond flour

- 2 Bananas

- 1 teaspoon of Salt

- 1 teaspoon of Sesame oil

- 1 tablespoon of Water

- Powdered sugar

Directions:

1. Peel the bananas. Dice into bite-size pieces.

2. In a bowl, combine the flour, salt, sesame oil. Add 1 tablespoon of water. Stir until combined in a smooth batter.

3. Dip banana in the batter. Set on a tray. Place the tray in the freezer for 10 minutes.

4. Cover bottom of the fryer with parchment paper. Spray parchment with oil.

5. Preheat fryer to 350 °F.

8. After that, stir in the mashed chickpeas. Cook for another 4 minutes or until thickened.

9. Serve along with microgreens. Place the greens at the bottom, followed by the scramble, and top it with cilantro or parsley.

Tip: if you don't prefer turmeric, you can omit it.

Nutrition: Calories 801 Kcal Proteins 41.5 g Carbohydrates 131.6 g Fat 14.7 g

10. Chocolate Breakfast Quinoa

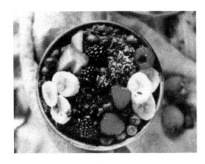

Preparation Time: 5 minutes

Cooking Time: 20 minutes

Servings: 1

Ingredients:

- ½ cup of Quinoa
- 1 ½ tablespoon of Cocoa
- 1 ½ cup of Soy Milk
- 1 ½ tablespoon of Maple Syrup
- 2 tablespoons of Peanut Butter
- Banana and strawberry slices (for topping)

Directions:

1. First, place the quinoa and soy milk into a medium-sized saucepan over medium-low heat.
2. After that, cook it for 13 to 15 minutes while keeping it covered.
3. Once the quinoa is cooked, stir in the peanut butter, sweetener, and cocoa powder to it.
4. Finally, transfer to a serving bowl.

Tip: instead of maple syrup, you can use brown rice syrup. You can even add cacao nibs to it. Also, you can add top to any berries.

Nutrition: Calories 650 Kcal Protein 19 g Carbohydrates 97 g Fat 22 g

11. Banana Quinoa Oatmeal

Preparation Time: 5 Minutes

Cooking Time: 10 Minutes

Servings: 1

Ingredients:

- ½ cup of Oats

- ½ cup of Quinoa, dry

- 2 Bananas, ripe

- ¾ cup of Almond Milk, light

- ½ teaspoon of Cinnamon, ground

- 2 tablespoons of Peanut Butter, organic

- 1 teaspoon of Vanilla

Directions:

1. To start, place the quinoa, oats, almond milk, cinnamon, and vanilla in a small saucepan.

2. Heat the saucepan over medium heat and bring the mixture to a boil.

3. Once it starts boiling, lower the heat and allow it to simmer for 10 to 15 minutes. Tip: the quinoa should have absorbed all the liquid at this time.

4. Next, fluff the quinoa mixture with a fork and then transfer to a serving bowl.

5. Now, spoon in the peanut butter and stir well.

6. Finally, top with the banana.

Tip: if you desire, you can add almonds to it for crunchiness.

Nutrition: Calories 386 Kcal Protein 11.7 g Carbohydrates 62.2 g

Fat 11.8 g

12. Avocado Sweet Potato Toast

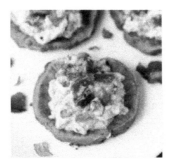

Preparation Time: 5 Minutes

Cooking Time: 10 Minutes

Servings: 1

Ingredients:

- 1 Sweet Potato, sliced into ¼-inch thick slices
- ½ of 1 Avocado, ripe
- ½ cup of Chickpeas
- 2 tablespoons of Sun-dried Tomatoes
- Salt & Pepper, as needed
- 1 teaspoon of Lemon Juice
- Pinch of Red Pepper
- 2 tablespoons of Vegan Cheese

Directions:

1. Start by slicing the sweet potato into five ¼-inch wide slices.
2. Next, toast the sweet potato in the toaster for 9 to 11 minutes.
3. Then, place the chickpeas in a medium-sized bowl and mash with the avocado.
4. Stir in the crushed red pepper, lemon juice, pepper, and salt.

5. Stir until everything comes together.

6. Finally, place the mixture onto the top of the sweet potato toast.

7. Top with cheese and sun-dried tomatoes.

Tip: if desired, you can add your choice of toppings.

Nutrition: Calories 452 Kcal Protein 19 g Carbohydrates 77 g Fat 11 g

13. Banana Strawberry Oats

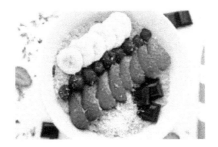

Preparation Time: 10 Minutes

Cooking Time: 20 Minutes

Servings: 1

Ingredients:

- ½ cup of Oats
- 1 cup of Zucchini, shredded
- 1 tablespoon of Almonds, sliced
- ½ teaspoon of Cinnamon
- ½ of 1 Banana, mashed
- 1 cup of Water
- ½ cup of Strawberries, sliced
- Dash of Sea Salt
- 1 tablespoon Flax Meal
- ½ scoop of Protein Powder

Directions:

1. First, combine oats, salt, water, and zucchini in a large saucepan.

2. Cook the mixture over medium-high heat and cook for 8 to 10 minutes or until the liquid is absorbed.

3. Now, spoon in all the remaining ingredients to the mixture and give everything a good stir.

4. Finally, transfer the mixture to a serving bowl and top it with almonds and strawberries.

5. Serve and enjoy.

Tip: you can use any berries instead of strawberries.

Nutrition: Calories 386 Kcal Proteins 23.7 g Carbohydrates 57.5 g Fat 8.9 g

14. Blueberry Banana Chia Oatmeal

Preparation Time: 10 Minutes

Cooking Time: 10 Minutes

Servings: 1

Ingredients:

- ¾ cup of Rolled Oats
- 1 cup of Plant Milk
- 2 tablespoons of Chia Seeds
- ¼ cup of Blueberries
- ½ cup of Water
- 2 tablespoons of Agave Syrup
- ½ teaspoon of Cinnamon
- 1 banana, ripe and mashed
- Dash of Sea Salt
- 1 teaspoon of Vanilla
- 2 tablespoons of Peanut Butter
- 1 ½ tablespoon of Water

Directions:

1. To begin with, combine the chia seeds, sea salt, cinnamon, and oats in a mason jar until mixed well.

2. Next, pour in the hemp milk along with the banana, vanilla, and water to the jar. Stir again.

3. Now, mix the peanut butter with water in a small mixing bowl for 2 to 3 minutes.

4. Tip: The mixture should be creamy in texture.

5. After that, pour the creamy mixture over the oats and stir.

6. Then, place the Mason jar in the refrigerator overnight.

7. Add your favorite topping (¼-cup of blueberries) and enjoy.

Tip: if you desire you can add coconut flakes and or cacao nibs as a topping.

Nutrition: Calories 864 Kcal Protein 23 g Carbohydrates 107.4 g Fat 42.1 g

15. Spinach Tofu Scramble

Preparation Time: 5 Minutes

Cooking Time: 10 Minutes

Servings: 2

Ingredients:

- 2 Tomatoes, finely chopped
- ¾ cup of Mushrooms, finely sliced
- ½ red bell pepper, finely chopped
- 10 ounces of Spinach
- 2 tablespoons of Olive Oil
- 1 teaspoon of Lemon Juice, freshly squeezed
- ½ teaspoon of Soy Sauce
- 2 Garlic cloves, minced
- Salt & Pepper, as needed
- 1 pound of Tofu, extra-firm & crumbled
- 1 avocado (optional)

Directions:

1. First, take a medium-sized skillet and heat it over medium-high heat.
2. Once the skillet becomes hot, spoon in the oil.
3. Next, stir in the tomatoes, red bell pepper, mushrooms, and garlic.
4. Cook them for 2 to 3 minutes or until softened.
5. Now, lower the heat to medium-low and spoon in the spinach, lemon juice, tofu, and soy sauce.

6. Mix well and cook for a further 8 minutes while stirring occasionally.

7. Then, check the seasoning and add salt and pepper as needed.

8. Serve it hot.

Tip: instead of spinach, you can substitute kale, chard, or asparagus. If you want, you can add avocado slices.

Nutrition: Calories 527 Kcal Protein 36 g Carbohydrates 43 g Fat 29 g

16. Hemp Seeds Oatmeal

Preparation Time: 10 minutes

Cooking Time: 0 minutes

Setting Time: 4 to 6 hours

Servings: 1

Ingredients:

- ¼ cup of Rolled Oats
- 1 tablespoon of Raisins
- ¼ teaspoon of Cinnamon
- 3 tablespoons of Hemp Seeds
- ½ cup of Soy Milk, unsweetened
- 1 tablespoon of Maple Syrup

Directions:

1. First, add all the ingredients to a large mason jar and mix well.
2. Now, place them in the refrigerator overnight.
3. Serve in the morning and enjoy.

Tip: to soften the raisins, you can soak them for a few hours.

Nutrition: Calories 364 Kcal Protein 19.1 g Carbohydrates 32.6 g Fat 19 g

17. <u>Gingerbread Chia Porridge</u>

Preparation Time: 10 minutes

Cooking Time: 15 minutes

Servings: 2 cups

Ingredients:

- ¼ cup of Chia Seeds
- Pinch of Clove, grounded
- ¾ cup of Soy milk, unsweetened
- ¼ teaspoon of Cinnamon, grounded
- 1 tablespoon of Maple syrup
- Dash of sea salt
- ¼ teaspoon of Ginger, grounded
- 1 tablespoon of Raisins, for garnishing

Directions:

1. Start by combining all the ingredients needed to make the oatmeal in a mason jar.
2. Place the Mason jar in the refrigerator for 8 hours.
3. Stir once the porridge before keeping it for refrigeration.
4. Now, garnish it with raisins.
5. Serve and enjoy.

Tip: you can also use chopped nuts for toppings.

Nutrition: Calories 307 Kcal Proteins 17.8 g Carbohydrates 36.6 g Fat 17.8 g

18. Banana Cauliflower Porridge

Preparation Time: 10 Minutes

Cooking Time: 15 Minutes

Servings: 1

Ingredients:

- 2 cups of Cauliflower Extract
- ¼ of 1 Pear
- ½ of 1 Banana, ripe
- 1 cup of Soy Milk, unsweetened
- ½ teaspoon of Vanilla Extract
- 1 ¼ teaspoon of Cinnamon
- 4 Strawberries
- 2 teaspoons of Maple Syrup
- ½ tablespoon of Almond Butter
- 1/8 teaspoon of Salt

Directions:

1. To make this nutritious oatmeal, place the cauliflower in the food processor and process until the cauliflower becomes riced or is in small granules.
2. Stir in the banana and mash it well.
3. After that, place the riced cauliflower-banana mixture into a small saucepan.
4. Heat the mixture over medium-high heat.

5. Next, spoon in all the remaining ingredients into the saucepan and give a good stir.

6. Lower the heat and cook for 14 minutes. Continue cooking until ready.

7. Place the oatmeal into a serving bowl and serve it immediately or warm.

Tip: you can even add sliced almonds to the mixture, or you can top it with berries and seeds.

Nutrition: Calories 351 Kcal Protein 15.1 g Carbohydrates 50.3 g Fat 12.1 g

19. Chai Flavored Quinoa

Preparation Time: 5 Minutes

Cooking Time: 20 Minutes

Servings: 1

Ingredients:

- ½ cup of Quinoa, washed
- ½ tablespoon of Coconut Palm Sugar
- 2 tablespoons of Chia Seeds
- 2 teaspoons of Maple Syrup
- 1 Chai Tea Bag
- 1 cup of Almond Milk, unsweetened

Directions:

1. To begin with, mix the quinoa with the almond milk and chai tea bag in a small saucepan.
2. Heat it over medium heat and bring the mixture to a boil.
3. Once it starts boiling, discard the chai bag.
4. Next, spoon in the coconut palm sugar and stir well.
5. Lower the heat and allow it to simmer for 18 to 20 minutes while keeping it covered.
6. Remove the saucepan from the heat. Set it aside for 10 minutes so that the quinoa absorbs all the liquid. Add chia seeds.
7. Finally, transfer the mixture to a serving bowl. Add maple syrup.
8. Serve immediately.

Tip: To enhance the flavor, you can add ground cinnamon to it.

Also, you can add sliced almonds to the mixture, or you can top it with berries and seeds.

Nutrition: Calories 383 Kcal Protein 13 g Carbohydrates 65.6 g Fat 8.7 g

LUNCH RECIPE

20. Mocha Smoothie

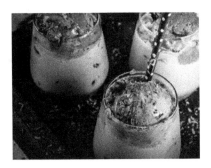

Preparation Time: 10 minutes

Cooking Time: 0 minutes

Servings: 3

Ingredients:

- 1 large avocado; peeled, pitted, and chopped roughly
- 3 tablespoons of cacao powder
- 2 teaspoons of instant coffee crystals
- 3 tablespoons of granulated Erythritol
- 1 teaspoon of organic vanilla extract
- ½ cup of heavy cream
- 1½ cup of unsweetened almond milk
- ½ cup of ice cubes

Directions:

1. In a high-speed blender, put all the ingredients and pulse until creamy.

2. Pour the smoothie into three glasses and serve immediately.

Nutrition: Calories 208 kcal Net Carbs 3.1 g Total Fat 19.9 g Saturated Fat 7.4 g Cholesterol 27 mg Sodium 101 mg Total Carbs 8.5 g Fiber 5.4 g Sugar 0.5 g Protein 2.9 g

21. Strawberry Smoothie

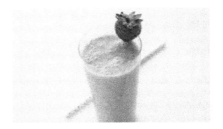

Preparation Time: 10 minutes

Cooking Time: 0 minutes

Servings: 2

Ingredients:

- ½ cup of fresh strawberries, hulled

- 8–10 fresh basil leaves

- 3–4 drops liquid stevia

- ½ cup of plain Greek yogurt

- 1 cup of unsweetened almond milk

- ¼ cup of ice cubes

Directions:

1. In a high-speed blender, put all the ingredients and pulse until creamy.

2. Pour the smoothie into two glasses and serve immediately.

Nutrition: Calories 72 kcal Net Carbs 4.8 g Total Fat 2.6 g Saturated Fat 0.7 g Cholesterol 5 mg Sodium: 115 mg Total Carbs 6.1 g Fiber: 1.3 g Sugar 3.5 g Protein 6.5 g

22. Breakfast Tacos

Preparation Time: 10 minutes

Cooking Time: 10 minutes

Servings: 4

Ingredients:

- 1 teaspoon of olive oil
- ½ sweet onion, chopped
- ½ red bell pepper, chopped
- ½ teaspoon of minced garlic
- 4 eggs, beaten
- ½ teaspoon of ground cumin
- Pinch red pepper flakes
- 4 tortillas
- ¼ cup of tomato salsa

Directions:

1. Warm-up oil in a large skillet on medium heat only. Add the onion, bell pepper, and garlic, and sauté until softened, about 5 minutes.

2. Add the eggs, cumin, and red pepper flakes, and scramble the eggs with the vegetables until cooked through fluffy.

3. Spoon one-fourth of the egg mixture into the center of each tortilla, and top each with 1 tablespoon of salsa. Serve immediately.

Nutrition: Calories 211 kcal Fat 7 g Sodium 346 mg Carbohydrates 17 g Phosphorus 120 mg Potassium 141 mg Protein 9 g

23. Mexican Scrambled Eggs in Tortilla

Preparation Time: 5 minutes

Cooking Time: 2 minutes

Servings: 2

Ingredients:

- 2 medium corn tortillas
- 4 egg whites
- 3 teaspoons of green chilies, diced
- ½ teaspoon of hot pepper sauce
- 2 tablespoons of salsa
- ½ teaspoon of salt

Directions:

1. Spray some cooking spray on a medium skillet and heat for a few seconds. Whisk the eggs with the green chilies, hot sauce, and comminute.

2. Add the eggs into the pan, and whisk with a spatula to scramble. Add the salt. Cook until fluffy and done (1-2 minutes) over low heat.

3. Open the tortillas and spread 1 tablespoon of salsa on each. Distribute the egg mixture onto the tortillas and wrap gently to make a burrito. Serve warm.

Nutrition: Calories 44.1 kcal Carbohydrate 2.23 g Protein 7.69 g Sodium 854 mg Potassium 189 mg Phosphorus 22 mg Fat 0.39 g

24. American Blueberry Pancakes

Preparation: 5 minutes **Cooking:** 10 minutes **Servings:** 6

Ingredients:

- 1 ½ cups of all-purpose flour, sifted
- 1 cup of buttermilk
- 3 tablespoons of sugar
- 2 tablespoons of unsalted butter, melted
- 2 teaspoons of baking powder
- 2 eggs, beaten
- 1 cup of canned blueberries, rinsed

Directions:

1. Combine the baking powder, flour, and sugar in a bowl. Make a hole in the middle, then slowly add the rest of the ingredients.
2. Begin to stir gently from the sides to the center with a spatula until you get a smooth and creamy batter. With cooking spray, spray the pan and place over medium heat.
3. Take one measuring cup and fill 1/3rd of its capacity with the batter to make each pancake.
4. Use a spoon to pour the pancake batter and let cook until golden brown. Flip once to cook the other side. Serve warm with optional agave syrup.

Nutrition: Calories 251.69 kcal Carbohydrate 41.68 g Protein 7.2 g Sodium 186.68 mg Potassium 142.87 mg Phosphorus 255.39 mg Fat 6.47 g

25. <u>Mocha Cereal</u>

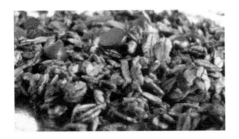

Preparation Time: 15 minutes

Cooking Time: 35 minutes

Servings: 4

Ingredients:

- ½ cup of golden flaxseeds meal
- ¼ cup of hemp seeds, hulled
- ¼ cup of hazelnut meal
- 1 tablespoon of cacao powder
- 3 packets of stevia
- ½ cup of cold-brewed coffee
- 1 tablespoon of butter, softened

Directions:

1. Preheat your oven to 300 °F.
2. Line a large baking sheet with a parchment paper.
3. In a high-speed blender, place the flaxseeds meal, hemp seeds, hazelnut meal, cacao powder, and stevia, and pulse until well combined.
4. Add the coffee, butter, and pulse for about 30 seconds more.

5. Place the mocha mixture onto the prepared baking sheet evenly and with the back of a spoon, press firmly to smooth the top surface.

6. Bake for approximately 15 minutes.

7. Now, set the temperature of the oven to 250 °F and bake for approximately 15 minutes more.

8. Remove the baking sheet from the oven and immediately with a pizza cutter, cut the mixture into bite-sized pieces.

9. Turn off the oven and place the baking sheet in the oven for at least 1 hour.

10. Remove the baking sheet from the oven and let the cereal cool completely before serving.

11. Serve with your favorite non-dairy milk and keto-friendly fruit.

Nutrition: Calories 201 kcal Net Carbs 2.6 g Total Fat 15 g Saturated Fat 3.4 g Cholesterol 8 mg Sodium: 21 mg Total Carbs 10 g Fiber7.4 g Sugar 0.2 g Protein 7.6 g

26. Raspberry Smoothie Bowl

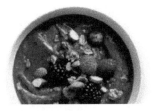

Preparation Time: 10 minutes

Cooking Time: 0 minutes

Servings: 3

Ingredients:

- 1 cup of frozen raspberries
- ¼ cup of collagen peptides
- ¼ cup of MCT oil
- 2 tablespoons of chia seeds
- 1 teaspoon of beet powder
- 1 teaspoon of organic vanilla extract
- drops of liquid stevia, to taste
- 1½ cups of unsweetened almond milk

Directions:

1. In a high-speed blender, put all the ingredients and pulse until smooth.
2. Transfer into 3 serving bowls and serve with your favorite topping.

Nutrition: Calories 238 kcal Net Carbs 4.1 g   Total Fat 22.4 g Saturated Fat 19 g Cholesterol 0 mg Sodium 202 mg Total Carbs 9 g Fiber 4.9 g Sugar 2 g Protein 11.1 g

27. Classic Western Omelet

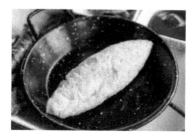

Preparation Time: 5 minutes

Cooking Time: 10 minutes

Servings: 1

Ingredients:

- 2 teaspoons of coconut oil

- 3 large eggs, whisked

- 1 Tablespoon of heavy cream

- Salt and pepper

- 1/4 cup of diced green pepper

- 1/4 cup of diced yellow onion

- 1/4 cup of diced ham

Directions:

1. In a small bowl, whisk the eggs, heavy cream, salt, and pepper.

2. Heat up 1 tsp. of coconut oil over medium heat in a small skillet.

3. Add the peppers and onions, then sauté the ham for 3 to 4 minutes.

4. Spoon the mixture in a cup, and heat the skillet with the remaining oil.

5. Pour in the whisked eggs & cook until the egg's bottom begins to set.

6. Tilt the pan and cook until almost set to spread the egg.

7. Spoon the ham and veggie mixture over half of the omelet and turn over.

8. Let cook the omelet until the eggs are set and then serve hot.

Nutrition: Calories 415 kcal Fat 232,5 g Protein 5 g Carbs 6,5 g Sugar 1,5 g Net Carbs 5 g

28. Nutty Pumpkin Smoothie

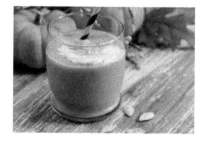

Preparation Time: 5 minutes

Cooking Time: None

Servings: 1

Ingredients:

- 1 cup of unsweetened cashew milk
- 1/2 cup of pumpkin puree
- 1/4 cup of heavy cream
- 1 tablespoon of raw almonds
- 1/4 teaspoon of pumpkin pie spice
- Liquid stevia extract, to taste

Directions:

1. Combine all the ingredients in a blender.
2. Press several times until the ingredients are thoroughly mixed
3. Pour into a large glass & enjoy immediately.

Nutrition: Calories 205 kcal Fat 16.5 g Protein 3 g Carbs 13 g Fiber 4.5 g Net Carbs 8.5 g

29. Broccoli, Kale, Egg Scramble

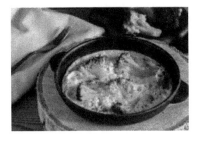

Preparation Time: 5 minutes

Cooking Time: 10 minutes

Servings: 1

Ingredients:

- 2 large eggs, whisked
- 1 tablespoon of heavy cream
- Salt and pepper
- 1 teaspoon of coconut oil
- 1 cup of fresh chopped kale
- 1/4 cup of frozen broccoli florets, thawed
- 2 tablespoons of grated parmesan cheese

Directions:

1. In a mug, whisk the eggs along with the heavy cream, salt, and pepper.
2. Heat 1 teaspoon of coconut oil over medium heat in a medium-size skillet.
3. Stir in the kale & broccoli, then cook about 1 to 2 minutes until the kale is wilted.
4. Pour in the eggs and cook until just set, stirring occasionally.

5. Stir in the cheese with parmesan and serve hot.

Nutrition: Calories 315 kcal Fat 23 g Protein 19.5 g Carbs 10 g Fiber 1.5 g Net Carbs 8.5 g

30. Greek Omelet

Preparation Time: 5 minutes

Cooking Time: 15 minutes

Servings: 2

Ingredients:

- 2 cups of fresh spinach leaves, chopped
- 2 green onions, white and green parts, sliced
- 4 large eggs
- ½ teaspoon of dried oregano
- 2 tablespoons of extra-virgin olive oil
- ½ cup of feta cheese, crumbled and divided
- ½ cup of grape tomatoes, halved
- ½ cup of sliced black or Kalamata olives

Directions:

1. Heat a large nonstick skillet over medium-low heat and toss in the spinach leaves and the white parts of the green onion.
2. Add a few teaspoons of water and cook, stirring frequently, for 8 to 10 minutes, or until the spinach leaves are wilted.
3. Transfer the spinach mixture to a bowl and set aside.
4. Remove the skillet from the heat and wipe with a paper towel.
5. While the spinach is cooking, break the eggs into a bowl and add the green parts of the green onions and the oregano. Beat lightly with a fork.
6. Return the skillet to the stove, add the olive oil, and turn up the heat to medium.

7. When the oil is hot, pour in the eggs and stir gently with the back of a fork for 30 seconds.

8. Cook for 2 to 3 minutes or until the eggs are almost set, loosening the edges occasionally with a spatula and gently tilting the skillet to let the uncooked eggs reach the surface of the skillet.

9. Add the spinach mixture, ¼ cup of feta cheese, grape tomatoes, and olives to the middle of the omelet. Let the eggs cook for another 20 to 30 seconds, until they're set.

10. Tap the handle of the pan sharply with your fist to loosen the omelet and then fold it over the spinach, cheese, tomatoes, and olives with a fork or spatula.

11. Slide the omelet onto a plate and scatter the remaining ¼ cup of feta cheese over top. Cut the omelet into two halves and serve immediately.

12. Substitution Tip: One (16-ounce) package of frozen chopped spinach can be used instead of fresh. Defrost first by running the frozen spinach under warm water in a strainer or microwaving for 1 to 2 minutes until the spinach is soft. Wrap a paper towel around the spinach and squeeze the excess water out over a sink.

Nutrition: Calories 422 kcal Total fat 36 g Total Carbs 9 g Fiber 3 g Sugar 4 g Protein 20 g Sodium 880 mg

31. Asparagus Cauliflower Tortilla

Preparation: 15 minutes **Cooking:** 15 minutes **Servings:** 4

Ingredients:

- 2 cup of asparagus, chopped into bite-size pieces
- 2 cup of cauliflower, chopped into bite-size pieces
- 1½ cup of onion, finely chopped
- 1 cup of liquid low cholesterol egg substitute
- 2 tablespoons of fresh parsley, finely chopped
- 2 teaspoons of olive oil
- Salt and freshly ground pepper
- ¼ teaspoon of dried thyme
- ¼ teaspoon of ground nutmeg
- 1 garlic clove, minced

Directions:

1. Place the asparagus and cauliflower in a dish with 1 tablespoon of water. Cook on high for around 3 to 5 minutes until tender but also crisp.
2. Sauté the onion in a skillet until translucent. Stir in the vegetables and remaining ingredients, and reduce the heat.
3. Cook within 10 to 15 minutes or until set and brown around the edges. Use a spatula to slide the tortilla onto a warm platter or serving plate. Slice into wedges and serve—delicious cold or reheated.

Nutrition: Calories 102 kcal Carbs 9 g   Fat 0 g Sodium 147.5 mg Protein 9 g Potassium 472 mg Phosphorous 97 mg

32. Toast Topped with Creamy Eggs

Preparation Time: 15 minutes

Cooking Time: 20 minutes

Servings: 2

Ingredients:

- 4 slices of white bread

- 6 eggs

- 4 ounces of Cream cheese

- 3 tablespoons of unsalted butter

- 1/3 cup of flour

- 1 1/2 cups of plain almond milk, unsweetened

- 1/2 tablespoons of Yellow mustard

- 1/8 teaspoon of Pepper

Directions:

1. Hard-boil the eggs for 12 minutes. Remove them from heat, drain and cover with cold water. Peel and chop boiled eggs. Put together the butter and flour in a saucepan at medium-low heat.

2. Mix until well combined. Add almond milk, cream cheese, mustard, and pepper to the butter and flour mixture. Let it thicken and add the eggs to the sauce, keeping at a warm heat.

3. Toast the bread and put the egg mixture over the toast before serving. Enjoy!

Nutrition: Calories 430 kcal Protein 15 g   Carbs 34 g   Fat 21 g Sodium 400 mg Potassium 250 mg Phosphorus 210 mg

33. Keto Cheese Tacos

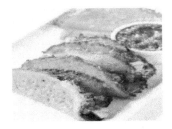

Preparation Time: 15 minutes

Cooking Time: 20 minutes

Servings: 6

Ingredients:

- 3 strips of bacon
- 1 oz. of cheddar cheese, shredded
- ½ avocado
- 2 tbsp. of butter
- 1 cup of mozzarella cheese, shredded
- 6 large eggs
- Salt and pepper, to taste

Directions:

1. Start by thoroughly cooking the bacon. Either in an oven for at least 15 to 20 minutes at 375°F or on the stovetop.
2. Heat a pan in a medium heat and add ⅓ cup of mozzarella.
3. Cook the cheese until it begins to bubble and turn brown on the side touching the pan. Pay close attention here!
4. Slip a spatula under the cheese and carefully unstick it from the pan.

5. Using a pair of tongs, drape the cheese over a wooden spoon that should be resting over a bowl or pot. Let the cheese to cool and form a taco shell shape.

6. Repeat Steps 2 to 5 with the remaining mozzarella.

7. Add the butter and eggs to the pan and cook thoroughly, adding salt and pepper to suit your taste.

8. Divide the eggs equally between your cheese shells.

9. Slice the avocado and divide the slices evenly between the tacos.

10. Chop or crumble your bacon, and divide equally between the tacos.

11. Sprinkle your cheddar cheese over the tops.

Nutrition Calories: 30Total Fat: 2.5gNet Carbs: 0.5gProtein: 1.5gFiber: 11.6g

34. Cheese Omelet

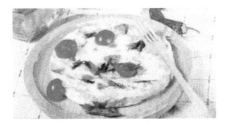

Preparation Time: 5 minutes

Cooking Time: 10 minutes

Servings: 2

Ingredients:

- 6 eggs
- 3 Ounces of ghee
- 7 ounces of shredded cheddar cheese
- salt and pepper

Directions:

1. Whisk the eggs until smooth. Compound half of the cheese and season it with salt and pepper.
2. Melt the butter in a pan. Pour in the mixture and let it sit for a few minutes (3-4)
3. When the mixture is looking good, add the other half of the cheese. Serve immediately.

Nutrition: Calories 897 kcal Carbs 4 g Fat 80 g Protein 40 g

35. Scrambled Eggs

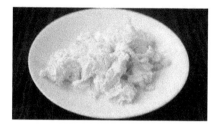

Preparation Time: 2 minutes

Cooking Time: 8 minutes

Servings: 4

Ingredients:

- 4 ounces of butter
- 8 eggs
- salt and pepper for taste

Directions:

1. Crack the eggs in a bowl, and whisk them together, while seasoning them.

2. Melt the butter in a skillet over medium heat, but don't turn it into brown.

3. Pour the eggs into the skillet and cook it for 1-2 mins, until they look and feel fluffy and creamy.

Tip: if you want to shake things up, you can pair this one up with bacon, salmon, or maybe avocado as well.

Nutrition: Calories 327 kcal Carbs 1 g Fat 31 g Protein 11 g

36. Almond Flour Pancakes

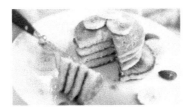

Preparation: 5 minutes **Cooking:** 5 minutes **Servings:** 4

Ingredients:

- ½ cup of almond flour
- ½ cup of cream cheese
- 2 medium eggs
- ½ teaspoon of cinnamon
- ½ teaspoon of granulated sweetener
- 1 teaspoon of grass-fed butter
- 1 tablespoon of sugar-free syrup

Directions:

1. Add all the ingredients into a blender and let them blend in well. Once done, set the batter aside.

2. On a non-stick pan at medium heat, fry pancakes with melted butter. Once the center starts to bubble, turn over. Once done with the pancake, move on to the rest, using the batter.

3. Finally, serve your pancakes warm, along with some low-carb fruit or with an exquisite side of sugar-free syrup to enjoy a healthy and tasty breakfast.

Nutrition: Calories 234 kcal Protein 11 g Fat 20 g Carbohydrates 4 g Fiber 1.5 g Net carbs 2.5 g

DINNER RECIPE

37. Savory Ham and Cheese Waffles

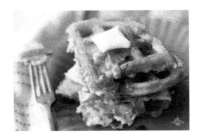

Preparation Time: 10 minutes

Cooking Time: 10 minutes

Servings: 2

Ingredients:

- 2 ounces (57 g) ham steak, chopped

- 2 ounces (57 g) Cheddar cheese, grated

- 8 eggs

- 1 teaspoon baking powder

- Basil, to taste

From the cupboard:

- 12 tablespoons butter, melted

- Olive oil, as needed

- 1-teaspoon sea salt

Special Equipment: A waffle iron

Directions:

1. Preheat the waffle iron and set aside.

2. Crack the eggs and keep the egg yolks and egg whites in two separate bowls.

3. Add the butter, baking powder, basil, and salt to the egg yolks. Whisk well. Fold in the chopped ham and stir until well combined. Set aside.

4. Lightly season the egg whites with salt and beat until it forms stiff peaks.

5. Add the egg whites into the bowl of egg yolk mixture. Allow to sit for about 5 minutes.

6. Lightly coat the waffle iron with the olive oil. Slowly pour half of the mixture in the waffle iron and cook for about 4 minutes. Repeat with the remaining egg mixture.

7. Take off from the waffle iron and serve warm on two serving plates.

Nutrition: Calories: 636 kcal Fat: 50.2g Protein: 45.1g Net carbs: 1.1g

38. Classic Spanakopita Frittata

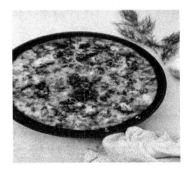

Preparation Time: 10 minutes

Cooking Time: 3-4 hours

Servings: 8

Ingredients:

- 12 eggs, beaten
- ½ cup feta cheese
- 1 cup heavy whipping cream
- 2 cups spinach, chopped
- 2 teaspoons garlic, minced

From the cupboard:

- 1 tablespoon extra-virgin olive oil

Directions:

1. Grease the bottom of the slow cooker, put with the olive oil lightly.

2. Stir together the beaten eggs, feta cheese, heavy cream, spinach, and garlic until well combined.

3. Slowly pour the mixture into the slow cooker. Cook covered on LOW for 3 to 4 hours, or until a knife inserted in the center comes out clean.

4. Take off from the slow cooker and cool for about 3 minutes before slicing.

Nutrition: Calories: 254 kcal Fat: 22.3g Protein: 11.1g Net carbs: 2.1g Fiber: 0g

39. Chicken Avocado Egg Bacon Salad

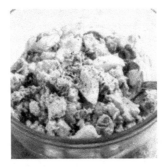

Preparation Time: 10 minutes

Cooking Time: 10 minutes

Servings: 4

Ingredients:

- 12 ounces of cooked chicken breast
- 6 slices of crumbled bacon
- 3 boiled eggs cut into cubes
- 1 cup of cherry tomatoes cut into halves
- 1/2 small sliced red onion
- 1 large avocado(s)
- 1/2 stick finely chopped celery

Salad Dressing:

- 1/2 cup of olive oil mayonnaise
- 2 tablespoons of sour cream
- 1 teaspoon of Dijon mustard
- 2 1/2 tablespoon of extra virgin olive oil
- 2 cloves minced garlic

- 2 teaspoons of lemon juice
- 4 cups of lettuce
- Salt and pepper to taste

Directions:

1. Combine all the ingredients together and mix them well for the salad dressing. Then, combine chicken, tomatoes, bacon, eggs, red onions, and celery together. Add about ¾ of the salad dressing and mix them well. Add the avocado and toss together gently. Check the taste and, if needed, add the remainder of the salad dressing as well. Finally, add salt, pepper to taste, and then serve it over lettuce.

Nutrition: Calories 387 kcal Fat 27 g Carbohydrates 2.5 g Fiber 1 g Net carbs 1.5 g Protein 24 g

40. Bacon Hash

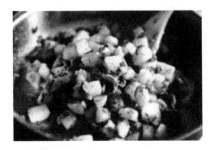

Preparation Time: 5 minutes

Cooking Time: 10 minutes

Servings: 2

Ingredients:

- 1 Small green pepper
- 2 Jalapenos
- 1 Small onion
- 4 Eggs
- 6 Bacon slices

Directions:

1. Chop the bacon into chunks using a food processor. Set aside for now. Slice the onions and peppers into thin strips. Dice the jalapenos as small as possible.

2. Heat a skillet and fry the veggies. Once browned, combine the fixings and cook until crispy. Place on a serving dish with the eggs.

Nutrition: Calories 366 kcal Carbohydrates 9 g Protein 23 g Fats 24 g

41. Nuts Porridge

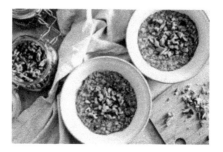

Preparation Time: 15 minutes

Cooking Time: 35 minutes

Servings: 5

Ingredients:

- ½ cup of pecans
- ½ cup of walnuts
- ¼ cup of sunflower seeds
- ¼ cup of chia seeds
- ¼ cup of unsweetened coconut flakes
- 1 ½ cups of unsweetened almond milk
- ½ teaspoon of ground cinnamon
- ¼ teaspoon of ground ginger
- 1 teaspoon of stevia powder
- 1 tablespoon of butter

Directions:

1. In a food processor, place the pecans, walnuts, and sunflower seeds, and pulse until a crumbly mixture is formed.

2. In a large pan, add the nuts mixture, chia seeds, coconut flakes, almond milk, spices, and stevia powder over medium heat, and bring to a gentle simmer, stirring frequently.

3. Adjust the heat to low and simmer for about 20–30 minutes, stirring frequently.

4. Remove from the heat and serve hot with the topping of butter.

Nutrition: Calories 289 kcal Net Carbs 2.8 g Total Fat 27.7 g Saturated Fat 6.1 g Cholesterol 6 mg Sodium 163 mg Total Carbs 8.9 g Fiber 6.1 g Sugar 1 g Protein 7.3 g

42. Egg Salad

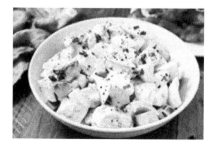

Preparation Time: 15 minutes

Cooking Time: 10 minutes

Servings: 4

Ingredients:

- 2 eggs

- 2 tablespoons of mayonnaise

- 1 teaspoon of Dijon mustard

- 1 teaspoon of lemon juice

- Salt and pepper to taste

- 4 Lettuce leaves

Directions:

1. In a medium saucepan, place the solid eggs gently.

2. Add some cold water so that the eggs are covered around an inch. Boil them for around 10 minutes.

3. Once done, remove them from the heat and let them cool. Peel the eggs while running them under cold water. Now add these to a food processor and pulse until they are chopped.

4. Add and stir mayonnaise, lemon juice, mustard, and salt and pepper. Ensure to taste and then adjust as necessary.

5. Finally, serve them with a few lettuce leaves and, if needed, bacon for wrapping.

Nutrition: Calories 222 kcal Fat 19 g Net carbs 1 g Protein 13 g

43. Fruited Curry Chicken Salad

Preparation Time: 45 minutes

Cooking Time: 0 minutes

Servings: 8

Ingredients:

- 4 cooked skinless and boneless chicken breasts
- 1 stalk of celery
- ½ cup of onion
- 1 medium-sized apple
- ¼ cup of seedless red grapes
- ¼ cup of seedless green grapes
- ½ cup of canned water chestnuts
- 1/8 teaspoon of black pepper
- ½ teaspoon of curry powder
- ¾ cup of mayonnaise

Directions:

1. Dice the chicken and chop the celery, onion, and apple. Also, drain and chop the water chestnuts.
2. Mix the chicken, celery, apple, grapes, onion, water chestnuts, pepper, curry powder, and mayonnaise in a large bowl. Toss all ingredients together, then serve or chill for later.

Nutrition: Calories 238 kcal Protein 14 g Carbohydrates 6 g Fat 18 g Sodium 162 mg Potassium 200 mg Phosphorus 115 mg

44. Rotini Pasta Salad

Preparation: 20 minutes **Cooking:** 10 minutes **Servings:** 8

Ingredients:

- 4 ounces of uncooked rotini pasta, uncooked
- 1-¼ of cups onion, chopped
- 4 large eggs
- 1 medium-sized cucumber, chopped
- ½ cup of mayonnaise
- ½ teaspoon of black pepper
- 1 tablespoon of dry mustard
- 1/3 teaspoon of salt (or exclude to reduce sodium)
- 1 teaspoon of prepared mustard
- ½ cup of sugar
- 1/3 cup of vinegar

Directions:

1. Cook the rotini based on the package's instruction directions, omit the salt, drain, and rinse. Hard boil the eggs, allow to cool, then peel

2. Combine and mix the rotini, onion, eggs, pepper, and cucumber in a large bowl. Combine the remaining ingredients to prepare the dressing.

3. Add the homemade dressing to the pasta. Mix properly. Put in the fridge to chill before you serve.

Nutrition: Calories 260 kcal Protein 6 g Carbohydrates 28 g Fat 14 g Sodium 193 mg Potassium 172 mg Phosphorus 87 mg

45. Capicola Egg Cups

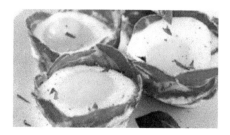

Preparation Time: 5 minutes

Cooking Time: 15 minutes

Servings: 4

Ingredients:

- 8 eggs
- 1 cup of cheddar cheese
- 4 ounces of Capicola or bacon (slices)
- salt, pepper, and basil to taste

Directions:

1. Preheat the oven to 400 °F. You will need 8 wells of a standard-size muffin pan.
2. Place the slices of bacon in the 8 wells, forming a cup shape. Sprinkle into each cup some of the cheese, according to your liking.
3. Crack an egg into each cup; season them with salt and pepper.
4. Bake for 10-15 mins. Serve hot, top it with basil.

Nutrition: Calories 171 kcal Carbs 1 g Fat 11 g Protein 16 g

46. BLT Party Bites

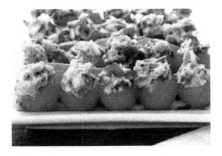

Preparation Time: 35 minutes

Cooking Time: 0 minute

Servings: 8

Ingredients:

- 4 ounces of bacon, chopped
- 3 tablespoons of panko breadcrumbs
- 1 tablespoon of Parmesan cheese, grated
- 1 teaspoon of mayonnaise
- 1 teaspoon of lemon juice
- Salt to taste
- ½ heart of Romaine lettuce, shredded
- 6 cocktail tomatoes

Directions:

1. Put the bacon in a pan over medium heat.
2. Fry until crispy.
3. Transfer bacon to a plate lined with a paper towel.
4. Add breadcrumbs and cook until crunchy.

5.   Transfer breadcrumbs to another plate also lined with a paper towel.

6.   Sprinkle Parmesan cheese on top of the breadcrumbs.

7.   Mix the mayonnaise, salt, and lemon juice.

8.   Toss the Romaine in the mayo mixture.

9.   Slice each tomato on the bottom to create a flat surface so it can stand by itself.

10. Slice the top off as well.

11. Scoop out the insides of the tomatoes.

12. Stuff each tomato with the bacon, Parmesan, breadcrumbs, and top with the lettuce.

Nutrition: Calories 107 kcal Total Fat 6.5 g Saturated Fat 2.1 g Cholesterol 16 mg Sodium 360 mg Total Carbohydrate 5.4 g Dietary Fiber 1.5 g Total Sugars 3.3 g Protein 6.5 g Potassium 372 mg

47. Bacon Wrapped Chicken Breast

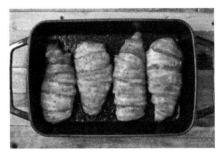

Preparation Time: 10 minutes

Cooking Time: 45 minutes

Servings: 4

Ingredients:

- 4 boneless, skinless chicken breast
- 8 ounces of sharp cheddar cheese
- 8 slices bacon
- 4 ounces of sliced jalapeno peppers
- 1 teaspoon of garlic powder
- Salt and pepper to taste

Directions:

1. Preheat the oven at around 350 °F. Ensure to season both sides of the chicken breast well with salt, garlic powder, and pepper. Place the chicken breast on a non-stick baking sheet (foil-covered). Cover the chicken with cheese and add jalapeno slices.

2. Cut the bacon slices in half and then place the four halves over each piece of chicken. Bake for around 30 to 45 minutes at

most. If the chicken is set but the bacon still feels undercooked, you may want to put it under the broiler for a few minutes. Once done, serve hot with a side of low-carb garlic parmesan roasted asparagus.

Nutrition: Calories 640 kcal Fat 48 g Carbohydrates 6 g Fiber 3 g Net carbs 3 g Protein 47 g

48. No-Bake Keto Power Bars

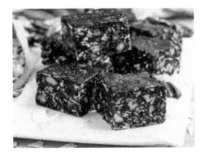

Preparation Time: 10 Minutes plus Overnight to Chill

Cooking Time: 20 minutes

Servings: 12 bars

Ingredients:

- ½ cup of pili nuts
- ½ cup of whole hazelnuts
- ½ cup of walnut halves
- ¼ cup of hulled sunflower seeds
- ¼ cup of unsweetened coconut flakes or chips
- ¼ cup of hulled hemp seeds
- 2 tablespoons of unsweetened cacao nibs
- 2 scoops of collagen powder (I use 1 scoop Perfect Keto vanilla collagen and 1 scoop Perfect Keto unflavored collagen powder)
- ½ teaspoon of ground cinnamon
- ½ teaspoon of sea salt
- ¼ cup of coconut oil, melted
- 1 teaspoon of vanilla extract

- Stevia or monk fruit to sweeten (optional if you are using unflavored collagen powder)

Directions:

1. Line a 9-inch square baking pan with parchment paper.
2. In a food processor or blender, combine the pili nuts, hazelnuts, walnuts, sunflower seeds, coconut, hemp seeds, cacao nibs, collagen powder, cinnamon, and salt and pulse a few times.
3. Add the coconut oil, vanilla extract, and sweetener (if using). Pulse again until the ingredients are combined. Do not over-pulse or it will turn to mush? You want the nuts and seeds to have some texture still.
4. Pour the mixture into the prepared pan and press it into an even layer. Cover with another piece of parchment (or fold over extra from the first piece) and place a heavy pan or dish on top to help press the bars together.
5. Refrigerate overnight and then cut into 12 bars. Store the bars in individual storage bags in the refrigerator for a quick grab-and-go breakfast.

Nutrition: Calories 242 kcal Total Fat 22 g Protein 6.5 g Total Carbs 4.5 g Fiber 2.5 g Net Carbs 2 g

49. Eggplant and Chives Spread

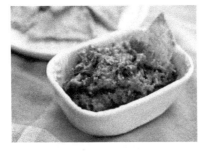

Preparation Time: 5 minutes

Cooking Time: 20 minutes

Servings: 4

Ingredients:

- 3 eggplants
- Salt and black pepper to the taste
- 2 tablespoons of chives, chopped
- 2 tablespoons of olive oil
- 2 teaspoons of sweet paprika

Directions:

1. Put the eggplants in your air fryer's basket and cook them for 20 minutes at 380 ° F.
2. Peel the eggplants put them in a blender, add the rest of the ingredients, pulse well, divide into bowls and serve for breakfast.

Nutrition: Calories 190 kcal Fat 7 g   Fiber 3 g Carbohydrates 5 g Protein 3 g

50. Cheddar and Broccoli Bake

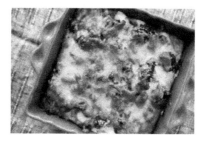

Preparation Time: 5 minutes

Cooking Time: 25 minutes

Servings: 4

Ingredients:

- 4 broccoli head, florets separated and roughly chopped
- 2 ounces of cheddar cheese, grated
- 4 eggs, whisked
- 1 cup of almond milk
- 2 teaspoons of cilantro, chopped
- Salt and black pepper to the taste

Directions:

1. In a bowl, put and mix the eggs with the milk, cilantro, salt, and pepper, and whisk.

2. Put the broccoli in your air fryer, add the eggs mix over it, spread, sprinkle the cheese on top, cook 350 ° F for 25 minutes, divide between plates and serve for breakfast.

Nutrition: Calories 214 kcal Fat 14 g Fiber 2 g Carbohydrates 4 g Protein 9 g

CONCLUSION

I
f you have fallen by the wayside, you'll be relieved to know you're
not alone. Even the most enthusiastic fitness guru struggles with
staying on course. If you have already missed a few steps, you can
start all over again and get it right this time.

Learn as many recipes as possible and prepare them for yourself in
order to better manage the ingredients being used. You can even do a
meal prep whereby you take one day to prepare the meals you wish to
eat during the coming week. This means even when you are too busy
or too tired to cook, all you have to do is get your prepped meal, warm
it, and enjoy a healthy meal. One reason to go for fast food is that it is
readily available.

Since intermittent fasting is not limiting what you can eat, there is a
wide variety to choose from these recipes. All you have to keep in
mind is the number of calories you are consuming per meal and this
cook have taken control of that. Meals that have low carbohydrate
content are ideal because they, in turn, have low caloric content as
well. Having more lean meats, fruits, and vegetables is ideal together
with grains too. If you're over the age of 50, then you know that your
metabolism slows down as time goes by. But in addition to that, you've
probably also noticed more and more weight gain. For many women
over 50, this is not only frustrating but downright discouraging - but it
doesn't have to be! Intermittent fasting for women over 50 is a very
popular topic because it does help curb some of the weight gain that
so many people are trying to avoid or work off. Intermittent fasting
for women over 50 can help you to work off the weight and also keep
your metabolism working at a healthy pace.

Here are some tips to help you get started on intermittent fasting for
women over 50. First of all, meal timing is not as important when it
comes to intermittent fasting for women over 50. For example, it's not
necessary to eat your meals within a two-hour window or anything like
that. It's much more important that you eat meals no less than three
times a day and that you make sure to eat at the same time each day.
It's very important to make sure that you're eating healthy meals.
Remember, the point of intermittent fasting for women over 50 is to
help you lose weight, not to give you an excuse to eat junk food! Try

to keep your meals low in carbohydrates and high in protein. You will lose weight much more quickly when you do this. In addition, it's also a good idea to eat smaller portions of vegetables with your meals - this is very important for maintaining a healthy body.

In addition to meal timing, you must also consider what you eat. Intermittent fasting for women over 50 is effective when it comes to weight loss. While it may not be the fastest way to lose weight, especially if you're a smaller person, it does work! If you combine intermittent fasting for women over 50 with a good exercise plan and healthy eating habits, then you'll have a much better chance of getting the weight off once and for all.

Finally, if you really want to be successful at intermittent fasting for women over 50, then it is important to get your hormones back in balance. In some cases, women may experience a weight loss plateau when they are in their 50's. This is not normal and it can be dangerous for your health if you don't address it soon. And in some cases, even when hormone levels are OK, you may still be dealing with pregnancy weight gain. This can be very discouraging. That's why it's so important to make sure you're not just limiting your intermittent fasting for women over 50 to when you eat, but also to how you're eating!

If you want to lose that extra weight that has been bothering you for so many years, then stop making excuses and start doing something about it! All it takes is a little information and the right kind of help. Most people who are overweight simply don't know how to properly do intermittent fasting for women over 50. Intermittent fasting for women over 50 lots of you are interested in intermittent fasting for women over 50, and even more you want to know exactly what it is. If you're looking for a fast weight loss plan that is easy to follow and is proven to work, then I would recommend an intermittent fasting diet. The reason why intermittent fasting diets work so well for weight loss is because it provides the body with adequate nutrients while also giving the body an energy source (calories) from the food that you eat.

Lightning Source UK Ltd.
Milton Keynes UK
UKHW020643010621
384724UK00004B/54